THE
ENERGY & WELL-BEING
POCKETBOOK

By Gillian Burn

Drawings by Phil Hailstone

"Good health and fitness are often taken for granted – a few simple steps can make a real difference to maintaining a happy and healthy life for the future. This pocketbook gives practical and clear advice, in an easily understood format. A few minutes' reading and following it will reduce the need to meet a doctor in the future."
Dr Steven Boorman, Chief Medical Adviser, Royal Mail Group

"This is a surprisingly thorough book, packed with practical advice. It will prove invaluable for anyone who wants to enjoy consistently high energy levels and the simple pleasure of feeling great."
Clive Lewis, Managing Director, Illumine Training

Published by:
Management Pocketbooks Ltd
Laurel House, Station Approach, Alresford, Hants SO24 9JH, U.K.
Tel: +44 (0)1962 735573   Fax: +44 (0)1962 733637
E-mail: sales@pocketbook.co.uk
Website: www.pocketbook.co.uk

This edition published 2004. Reprinted 2005, 2007.

© Gillian Burn 2004.

British Library Cataloguing-in-Publication Data – A catalogue record for this book is available from the British Library.

ISBN 978 1 903776 09 4

Design, typesetting and graphics by **efex ltd**. Printed in U.K.

CONTENTS

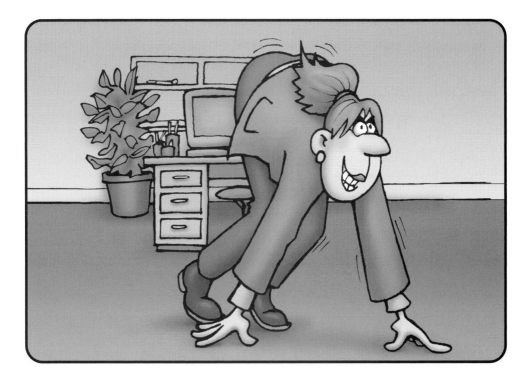

1NTRODUCTION

WHAT IS ENERGY?

Energy is essential for good health to nourish our bodies and minds.
We all need sufficient stores of energy every day to:

- Feel good
- Achieve what we want to achieve
- And enjoy each day to the full

If your energy is low you may feel lethargic, unhappy, lazy, tired, under pressure, not wanting to wake up in the mornings.

If your energy levels are high you may be smiling, happy, cheerful, able to complete tasks, raring to go, feeling full of vitality and vigour.

WHAT IS ENERGY?

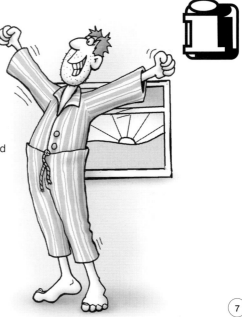

- Health
- Vitality
- Raring to go
- Waking early and jumping out of bed
- Zest for life
- Power
- Strength
- Endurance
- Personal achievement
- Dynamism

What else does energy mean for you?

WHAT YOU NEED TO BE ENERGETIC

- Fuel from food and water which is stored in your body cells, muscles and liver, before being converted to energy
- Adequate rest and sleep
- A healthy environment around you
- Sufficient exercise and activity
- Variety and challenge in your work and play
- Supportive people around you

Add to the list anything else that you think you need.

UNDERSTANDING ENERGY ZAPPERS

WHAT DRAINS YOUR ENERGY?

- Time of the day - are there times in the day when your mind doesn't seem so clear and you are not working as productively, eg early afternoon?
- Season - are you more lethargic in the winter than in the spring?
- Food and drink - do certain foods make you feel sleepy, eg roast Sunday lunch or a glass or two of wine?
- Activity and exercise - do you feel less and less energetic the less you do?
- Sleep - after a poor night's sleep, do you find it hard to get going and harder to complete jobs during the day?
- During illness - do you sleep more and have less energy whilst your body is recovering from an illness?
- Under stress - do you feel energy draining from you?

Things that drain my energy	Their effect
Travel	Makes me tired
Winter	Makes me irritable and lethargic
Late nights	Give me dull skin

THE ENERGY CHOICE FOR YOU

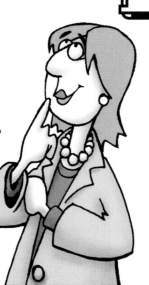

Consider what you personally need to feel energetic:

- How do you want to feel?
- What do you need to help you?
- What will you look like when you are energetic?
- What will your inner voice say about your energy?
- How will people describe your energy to others?

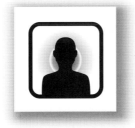

THE ENERGY FACTOR

THE ENERGY FACTOR

ENERGY AND WELL-BEING AUDIT

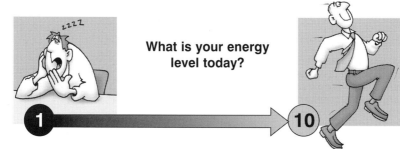

What is your energy level today?

Give yourself a score from one to ten for your own personal energy level:

1   feeling very lazy, like *Slowpoke Rodrigues* or a couch potato
10   full of energy, like *Speedy Gonzales* or Mr. Fit

Now consider how energetic you would like to feel.

UNDERSTANDING YOUR BODY CLOCK

The body clock relates to times of the day that you may feel more like doing certain activities. Our bodies have natural body rhythms and biorhythms which can affect us.

Some of us are at our best in the morning, waking early and preferring to start tasks early in the day, often described as 'larks'. Other people struggle to get started in the morning and are happier in the afternoon and evening, and may even work late into the night. These are known as 'owls'.

It is useful to understand whether you are more like a lark or an owl and to choose your optimum times of the day to perform certain tasks or projects.

Our bodies also have natural 'highs' and 'lows' during the day, linked to the action of hormones (adrenaline) and temperature control.

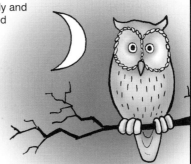

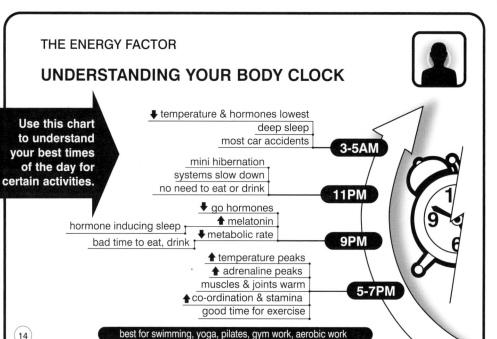

THE ENERGY FACTOR

UNDERSTANDING YOUR BODY CLOCK

Use this chart to understand your best times of the day for certain activities.

⬇ temperature & hormones lowest
deep sleep
most car accidents
3-5AM

mini hibernation
systems slow down
no need to eat or drink
11PM

⬇ go hormones
⬆ melatonin
hormone inducing sleep
⬇ metabolic rate
bad time to eat, drink
9PM

⬆ temperature peaks
⬆ adrenaline peaks
muscles & joints warm
⬆ co-ordination & stamina
good time for exercise
5-7PM

best for swimming, yoga, pilates, gym work, aerobic work

THE ENERGY FACTOR

UNDERSTANDING YOUR BODY CLOCK

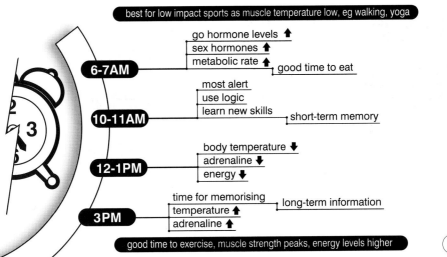

best for low impact sports as muscle temperature low, eg walking, yoga

6-7AM
- go hormone levels ↑
- sex hormones ↑
- metabolic rate ↑ — good time to eat

10-11AM
- most alert
- use logic
- learn new skills — short-term memory

12-1PM
- body temperature ↓
- adrenaline ↓
- energy ↓

3PM
- time for memorising — long-term information
- temperature ↑
- adrenaline ↑

good time to exercise, muscle strength peaks, energy levels higher

THE ENERGY FACTOR

UNDERSTANDING YOUR BODY CLOCK
WHAT ARE BIORHYTHMS?

- Biorhythms are natural body clocks triggered from the hypothalamus in the brain in response to light, and are genetically determined
- Timings vary from person to person
- They depend on month, seasons, hormones, heartbeat, respiration and temperature
- They affect physical, emotional and intellectual performance

Be aware of your *energy* times. Your energy may be increased during the full moon, during spring, at certain times of the month linked to female hormone levels, in cool or hot weather, etc.

MIND/BODY CONNECTION

How you feel in your mind will also affect how energetic you feel. How you look on the outside and how you feel inside are reflections of your subconscious mind. The mind and body are one system; what you think about affects your body!

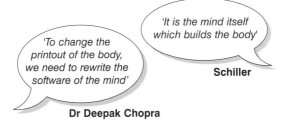

'It is the mind itself which builds the body'

Schiller

'To change the printout of the body, we need to rewrite the software of the mind'

Dr Deepak Chopra

(17)

CREATING ENDORPHINS

Endorphins are called the 'Elixir of Life'.

They are biochemicals, discovered in the 1970s and are chemically similar to opium and morphine, but 1000 times stronger.

Endorphins:

- Are not addictive or damaging
- Are naturally produced in the body
- Create physical pleasure and kill pain
- Help to heal wounds and disease
- Boost the immune system
- Create feelings of well-being, euphoria and bliss!

We can create natural endorphins in our bodies using the simple steps outlined on the next page.

CREATING ENDORPHINS

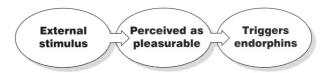

- Think of a lovely experience!
- PAUSE and enjoy the memory
- Allow the positive feelings to flow into your body and breathe into your muscles

To help unlock endorphins within your body, think of a lovely experience, perhaps a favourite holiday, a beautiful beach, a tranquil garden, or a special moment. Create your own list of positive triggers which are personal to you. As you pause and stop what you are doing to enjoy the memory, the positive hormones, endorphins, will flow through your body. Find time each day to pause for a moment and focus on one or two of your own positive triggers to allow the endorphin effect to occur, eg when you are waiting in a queue, at red traffic lights or on your journey to or from work.

Use the list on the next page to highlight your positive triggers.

POSITIVE THOUGHTS

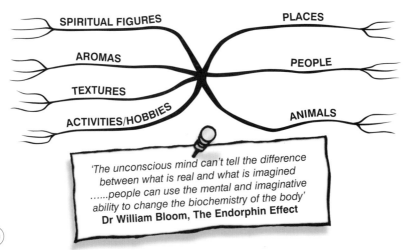

SPIRITUAL FIGURES

PLACES

AROMAS

PEOPLE

TEXTURES

ACTIVITIES/HOBBIES

ANIMALS

'The unconscious mind can't tell the difference between what is real and what is imagined ......people can use the mental and imaginative ability to change the biochemistry of the body'
Dr William Bloom, The Endorphin Effect

THE ENERGY FACTOR

SLEEP – ARE YOU GETTING ENOUGH?

We spend about a third of our lives asleep and most of us need between six and eight hours sleep to be alert and effective throughout the day.

Adequate sleep is important to ensure we have sufficient energy. However, it is also essential to help restore normal function in the body.

During sleep the following processes occur:

- Our cells recharge and assimilate information from the day
- Physical energy is renewed
- Growth hormones help repair and rebuild cells and tissues, eg skin repair
- Muscular energy is replenished
- Immune system works to combat illness
- The body enjoys a deep form of rest

Your sleeping pattern will be adversely affected by sedentary behaviour, lack of a regular sleep pattern and the use of stimulants, eg coffee, alcohol or nicotine.

SNOOZING SOLUTIONS

GOLDEN RULES FOR GOOD SLEEP

1. Establish a bedtime routine, with regular times for going to bed and getting up.
2. Sleep only as much as you need to feel well rested and wake up feeling refreshed.
3. Get up at the same time every day – lying in on days off disrupts sleep patterns. Taking a 10 - 20 minute afternoon power nap is a better option for your body!
4. Make your bedroom quiet and relaxing; reduce unwanted noise and light. Invest in a good mattress and pillows, and keep the room cool.
5. Don't go to bed hungry – carbohydrates have a mild sleep-enhancing effect, so try toast, cereal or some fruit. Large meals close to bedtime are hard to digest; keep to light snacks and avoid sugary, spicy or fatty foods which act as stimulants.
6. Avoid drinks containing caffeine (coffee, some teas, colas and chocolate).
7. Early evening exercise will promote sleep; your body temperature rises and later falls, making it easier to sleep. Try not to exercise too close to bedtime (within 2 – 3 hours).
8. Consider relaxation techniques, eg: deep breathing, relaxing each limb in your body, visualisation, aromatherapy oils (lavender, ylang ylang), drinking herb teas (camomile).
9. If you wake at night, get up, do something relaxing in another room (jigsaws are recommended!) and then return to bed later.

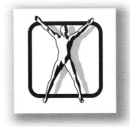

EXERCISE FOR ENERGY

EXERCISE FOR ENERGY

EVERYDAY ACTIVITY

We have over 1,000 moving parts in our bodies – but do we regularly move them? Our bodies are designed to move, yet seven out of ten people do not take enough exercise to benefit their health.

Statistics from The British Heart Foundation National Centre for Physical Activity and Health show that only 37% of men and 25% of women are active enough to benefit their health, but 80% think they are! *(Allied Dunbar Fitness Survey)*

70% of women and 63% of men across all ages participate in less than the recommended level of physical activity. *(Joint Health Survey, 1999)*

An inactive lifestyle has a substantial negative effect on individual health. *(Department of Health, 2004)*

People over the age of 50 are at a much greater risk of heart disease, but only 30% of 50-64 year olds are active enough to safeguard their health. (www.bhf.org.uk and www.bhfactive.org.uk)

EXERCISE FOR ENERGY

HOW ACTIVE ARE YOU?

Ask yourself the following questions and ✓ which is most like you:

	Exercise behaviour which best suits you	Example of behaviour	✓
1.	I do not exercise and I do not intend to start	Couch potato 'Mr. Procrastinator' No time	☐
2.	I do not exercise but I am thinking of starting	I'm thinking about it I belong to a gym, but haven't been yet!	☐
3.	I exercise once in a while but not regularly	I prefer fine weather 'Mrs. Occasional' It depends on my friends	☐
4.	I exercise regularly but started only recently	I swim at weekends and now walk to the station daily	☐
5.	I exercise regularly (and have done for at least six months)	I feel really good and have more energy	☐

Where you choose to mark yourself provides a useful benchmark. Whatever your score, consider what you could do to move to the next number in your exercise behaviour.

EXERCISE FOR ENERGY

HOW MUCH EXERCISE IS ENOUGH?

To create energy in your body, follow the easy formula recommended by both the Department of Health and The British Heart Foundation.

Aim to exercise for: **30 M**inutes
Most days
Moderate intensity

- 30 minutes - can be in five to ten minute slots throughout the day

- Most days - at least five times each week

- Moderate activity - so you breathe a little faster, feel warmer and have a slightly faster heart beat. The intensity should be comfortable and you should still be able to talk!

- Exercise you enjoy, eg walking, cycling, dancing or swimming

Remember, you can include playing with children, housework, gardening, DIY, and so on. It all counts towards your 30 minutes of activity.

CREATING ACTIVE HABITS

BURN EXTRA CALORIES

Compare activities on the following chart:

Home activities	Calories used per 30 mins
Vacuuming	120
Washing the car	120
Gardening	144
Playing with children	110
Active shopping	96

Home activities	Calories used
Phone call	
- sitting	5
- standing	10
10 minute walk	100
Take lift	5
Walk up 3 flights	35
Park next to entrance	5
Park at far end of car park	25
30 minute office meeting	30
30 minute walking meeting	150

Leisure activities	Calories used per 30 mins
Dancing	160
Ball games	200
Racquet games	240
Swimming	345
Dog walking	170

BENEFITS OF EXERCISE

By exercising for just 30 minutes you bring about the following benefits:

- Increase your energy and stamina
- Increase the oxygen supply to your brain, improving brain function (a well exercised body has 500 mls. more blood and the brain uses 25% of circulating blood)
- Improve muscle and lung function
- Keep your heart fit and strong
- Help to manage weight, blood pressure, cholesterol and blood sugar levels
- Help release 'happy hormones' to reduce stress, create relaxation and improve how you feel
- Help you look and feel better, improving your self-esteem and self-confidence

BENEFITS OF WALKING

If you are not sure where to start, remember that walking is described as one of the best forms of exercise.

So, why is walking so good? It's healthy, cheap, easy, low risk and available to most people.

- Most people can join in
- No special equipment required
- Low impact
- You can build up the daily amount
- Many health gains
- Quick results
- Not age- or cost-related

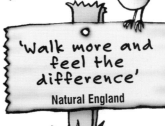

'Walk more and feel the difference'

Natural England

BENEFITS OF WALKING

When you walk you use over 250 muscles and walking just two miles a day can reduce the risk of a heart attack by 28%. Walking this distance can reduce the risk of developing type 2 diabetes and can reduce weight by as much as 14 lbs (6 kgs) in three months.

At any pace, walking will help to:

- Increase good cholesterol
- Improve muscle strength
- Reduce weight
- Improve mental health
- Benefit immune system and reduce bowel cancer
- Prevent development of osteoarthritis and osteoporosis in certain groups

At a brisk pace, walking will:

- Reduce blood pressure
- Improve functioning of heart and lungs

A person weighing 62kg walking a mile in 20 minutes will burn five calories per minute = 100 calories.

EXERCISE FOR ENERGY

BENEFITS OF WALKING

Frequency   Aim to walk on five or more days each week

Intensity   Moderate

Time   Initially 3 x 10-minute sessions or 2 x 15-minute sessions, building up to 1 continuous session of 30 minutes

Remember, every little bit counts - start where you are and build up gently.

During an average day we may walk 5,000 -7,000 steps; the aim is to walk at least 10,000 every day. Try using a pedometer to see how far you walk each day.

Ref: BHF, Natural England, Walking the Way to Health (www.whi.org)
Be-Active Ltd (www.be-activeltd.co.uk)

EXERCISE FOR ENERGY

ENERGY BREAKS

Our bodies need regular breaks during the day, at least every 45 minutes. This is a time for physical movement and a change of visual field, especially if you sit at a computer throughout the day. You can achieve this simply by getting up to get a glass of water, or taking some 'brain breaks' during your busy day.

Regular breaks help the brain assimilate information by increasing the blood supply to the brain and changing perspective on a situation.

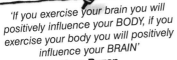

'If you exercise your brain you will positively influence your BODY, if you exercise your body you will positively influence your BRAIN'
Tony Buzan

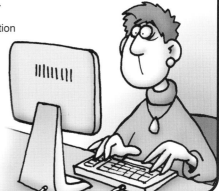

EXERCISE FOR ENERGY

BRAIN BREAK DESK EXERCISES

Try the following exercises adapted from The Chartered Society of Physiotherapy:

- **Executive stretch or elbow flare** - place your hands behind your neck loosely grasped. Keep your head and neck tall. Squeeze below the shoulder blades and take your elbows back, taking care not to press on your neck. Hold for five seconds.
- **Shoulder shrug** - keep your shoulders back and lift them towards your ears, breathing in slowly. Tighten the muscles in your shoulders and hold for five seconds. Breathe out as you drop the shoulders. Repeat three times.
- **Monkey stretch** - lift your right arm up by your right ear and stretch to the ceiling, then gently place your right hand by your left ear, over the top of your head. Repeat on the left side, by gently stretching your left arm up by your left ear and up towards the ceiling, then gently place your left hand by your right ear, over the top of your head.

BRAIN BREAK DESK EXERCISES

- ***T junction*** - stretch both arms out by your sides, level with your shoulders, so your body creates a T position. Move your right arm in a small circle clockwise and your left arm in a small circle anticlockwise and then change direction in both arms.

- ***Eye relaxation*** - look ahead and imagine a clock face. Move your eyes slowly clockwise keeping your head still, briefly stopping at 3pm, 6pm, 9pm and 12pm. Then reverse, moving your eyes anticlockwise, stopping briefly at 9pm, 6pm and 3pm and back to 12pm.

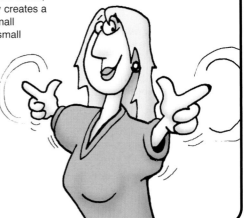

EXERCISE FOR ENERGY

ACTIVE ZONE

FOUR PILLARS

Consider the following activity ideas to create body awareness from the inside out, improve your posture and poise, and increase your flexibility of movement.

Keeping your body tuned - four pillars
The four pillars to help keep your body tuned are: poise and posture, aerobic exercise, flexibility and muscular strength.

1. Poise and posture
To maintain correct alignment of the skeletal system.

- Ensures bones and muscles work efficiently
- Maintains muscle balance
- Provides even weight distribution
- Promotes fluidity of movement - watch how a cat or a young child moves!

Three ways to improve your posture:
1. Consider how you stand
2. Try the Pilates relaxation position when lying down to relax (see page 40 onwards)
3. Think about your position when sitting at your desk

ACTIVE ZONE

FOUR PILLARS (Cont'd)

2. Aerobic exercise

Aerobic exercise is an important component to achieve overall fitness. Your heart beats faster, you feel warmer and you will be pumping more oxygen around your body as your breathing rate also increases.

Aerobic exercise can be achieved through gentle jogging, swimming, brisk walking, some sports, etc.

What are the benefits?

- Improves size, strength and pumping efficiency of the heart
- Strengthens breathing muscles
- Tones up muscles throughout body
- Increases the total amount of blood circulating
- Promotes physical fitness
- Promotes mental fitness to help with planning, organising, and juggling different tasks and intellectual challenges

ACTIVE ZONE

FOUR PILLARS (Cont'd)

3. Flexibility

This is the ability of your muscles to work through their full range of movement. Pilates and yoga exercises both help to increase the body's flexibility. Flexibility exercises are also a key component during exercise to help stretch muscles gently in the warm up phase and finally to help lengthen muscles in the cool down phase.

By improving flexibility you will:

- Improve the nervous system by increasing the flow of nerve messages
- Enhance oxygen flow around body
- Provide fluidity of movement around the joints
- Create flexibility of mind as well as body

EXERCISE FOR ENERGY

ACTIVE ZONE

FOUR PILLARS (Cont'd)

4. Muscular strength

Muscular strength refers to the ability of the body and muscle system to lift, pull, push and rotate. By maintaining muscular strength we help to:

- Tone muscles
- Strengthen bones
- Improve functional ability

As we get older we experience a gradual loss of muscle, mainly caused by an increasingly sedentary lifestyle. The results are:

- Increase in body fat, decline in aerobic capacity and vitality
- Decline in blood sugar tolerance, increasing insulin resistance interfering with the body's ability to produce energy
- Loss of bone density, increasing susceptibility to osteoporosis
- Slowing of metabolism

The good news is that with exercise and strength training, the decline can be reversed regenerating muscle mass and rejuvenating the body.

EXERCISE FOR ENERGY

ACTIVE ZONE
ACTIVITIES TO DEVELOP YOUR STRENGTH

1 Upper body

Press ups (to tone arms). Face the floor, hands under shoulders. Lower body towards floor until arms are at 90 degrees. Return to starting position.

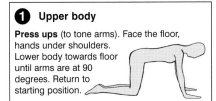

2 Lower back

Angels (to strengthen back). Lie prone. Lift opposite arm and leg just off floor.

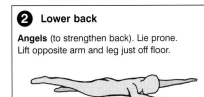

3 Mid body

Sit ups with feet on chair (to flatten stomach). Hands behind head. Lift chin onto chest, draw tummy in.

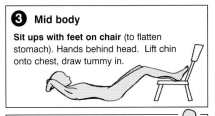

4 Legs

Squats (to tone legs). Feet hip width apart, bend knees to 90 degrees, allow body to lean forward until it is at right angles to thighs.

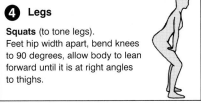

EXERCISE FOR ENERGY

PILATES

Pilates is a form of exercise and body conditioning. It is a complete and thorough method of physical conditioning. The exercises are gentle yet effective, and suitable for all ages and all people. It is also highly recommended by physiotherapists, osteopaths and chiropractors.

Joseph Pilates (born 1880) designed the original exercises to improve his own health, fitness and body image. The Pilates Method has grown rapidly throughout the world and is now taught in many centres.

Pilates will help you:

- Get into shape and tone up
- Improve your posture
- Ease and prevent back problems
- Get fit for sport
- Just relax and de-stress

EXERCISE FOR ENERGY

PILATES

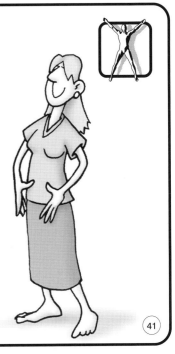

Pilates works on core stability by targeting the deep postural muscles and building strength from inside out. It also builds muscle tone throughout the body, helps to strengthen weak muscles, lengthen short muscles and increase joint mobility. It focuses on correct alignment so that all your vital organs are properly supported, enabling them to function efficiently.

Pilates has a positive effect on general health and, with the focus on breathing, helps to stimulate the circulatory system, oxygenating the blood, aiding lymphatic drainage and releasing endorphins (happy hormones) to make you feel good.

EXERCISE FOR ENERGY

PILATES

Pilates incorporates eight principles:

1. Relaxation: relaxing into movements
2. Concentration: maintaining control for correct movement
3. Alignment: maintaining correct placement so vital organs are properly supported
4. Breathing: wide and full into the chest, breathing in to prepare for movement and breathing out as you move
5. Co-ordination: developing a sense of body awareness to refine movements
6. Flowing movements: to allow muscles to lengthen from a strong centre
7. Stamina: slowly increasing stamina and endurance
8. Centring: creating a strong centre around the abdominal muscles, referred to as a 'girdle of strength'

'In 10 sessions you'll feel the difference, in 20 you'll see the difference, and in 30 you'll have a new body.'

Joseph Pilates

PILATES

Pilates has been described as:

> 'The thinking person's exercise: a safe and comprehensive method for relieving and preventing chronic back problems.'

Andrew Ferguson, osteopath

> 'Pilates is the single, most effective exercise technique I have ever known.'

Stephanie Powers, actress

> 'Pilates is a total joy ... I felt taller, leaner and fitter ... Pilates seems safe and effective.'

Family Circle Magazine

Ref: The Body Control Pilates Association, 2007

PILATES

EXERCISES: RELAXATION POSITION

Try the following exercises to get you started:

Relaxation position
Also called the *semi-supine* position in Alexander Technique or *Constructive Rest* position.

This exercise helps to develop body awareness, lengthens the spine and releases any areas where there may be tension. It enables the body to release tensions and tight muscles in a gravity-reduced way.

- Lie on your back with your knees gently bent, feet flat on the floor hip-width apart and parallel
- Place a small, firm pillow under your head to allow gravity to lengthen the neck
- Rest your hands gently on your abdomen
- Become aware of the lower back releasing into the floor
- Try to release the upper back into the floor by softening the breastbone and the front of the shoulders, allow the shoulders to 'melt' into the floor
- Your neck is naturally long with the top of your head lengthening away, jaw relaxed
- Gently breathe wide into the chest

PILATES

EXERCISES: RELAXATION POSITION

Your neck can lengthen and release.

Your lower back can release.

Your thighs can release. The hips can open.

EXERCISE FOR ENERGY

PILATES
EXERCISES: CORKSCREW

This exercise releases tightness and tension in the shoulders and arms, often caused by long hours at a desk! It also helps to release any neck tension.

- Stand with feet firmly on the ground
- Breathe in to prepare and lengthen through the spine
- Breathe out as you allow your arms to float upwards, keeping your shoulders relaxed
- Gently clasp your hands behind your head
- As you breathe in, shrug your shoulders up to your ears
- Breathe out as you drop your shoulders down
- Breathe in to gently bring your elbows back a little and your shoulder blades will come together
- Breathe out to release your hands and slowly bring them back to your side, opening them wide
- Allow your head, neck and spine to lengthen up as the arms come down, picturing a corkscrew

PILATES

EXERCISES: CORKSCREW

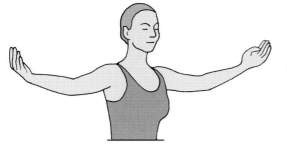

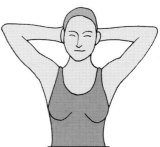

EXERCISE FOR ENERGY

YOGA

Yoga originated in India several thousand years ago. The word 'yoga' means the union of the body, mind and spirit. There are now many forms of yoga with the focus on balancing the mind and body by performing a series of postures, breathing techniques and relaxation. The posture exercises aim to convert negative, sluggish energy into positive energy and a sense of health and vitality.

Yoga will help to:

- Detoxify the body by speeding up the removal of waste and unwanted toxins
- Define body shape
- Increase flexibility
- Develop suppleness, strength and stamina

Yoga exercises can be performed on your own or within a class. A yoga programme will often incorporate meditation allowing complete relaxation of the mind and body.

EXERCISE FOR ENERGY

YOGA

SALUTE TO THE SUN

The 'Salute to the Sun' posture incorporates several movements in one exercise. The beauty of the exercise is that it can take as little as five minutes if you complete the exercise just once, or if you have more time available you can repeat the exercise six to eight times, slowly increasing the movement in the body.

The movements create a sequence of positions which help to stretch all the major muscle groups, promoting flexibility in the limbs and mobility in the spine. The exercise works on both the mind and body by regulating breathing and relaxing and focusing the mind.

Try it as a morning stretch before you start your day. All the movements are made on the out breath, keeping the sequence of movements relaxed and flowing. Throughout the exercise your shoulders should feel relaxed and your hips should move freely without tension.

EXERCISE FOR ENERGY

YOGA
EXERCISE: SALUTE TO THE SUN

1. Stand with your hands in the prayer position, thumbs against the sternum

2. Inhale and swing arms back above your head, arching your back gently

3. Exhale and come into a forward bend, bringing your hands as near to the floor as is comfortable for you. Relax your head down towards the floor

4. Take your right foot back into a lunge with your hips down. Arms beside your body and look up

5. Keep your hands shoulder-width apart and go into the 'dog pose'

6. Drop your knees, chest and chin to the floor

7. Push up through the 'cobra'

8. Go back into the 'dog pose'

9. Bring your right foot forward into the lunge position with arms beside your body

10. Step forward into the forward bend again (Step 3)

11. Come up into standing position (taking care to raise your head slowly to prevent feeling light headed). Gently arch your back slightly

12. Finish bringing your hands back into the prayer position, feet apart and take a deep breath in and out, before repeating the sequence to the other side (with the left foot leading)

EXERCISE FOR ENERGY

YOGA

EXERCISE: SALUTE TO THE SUN

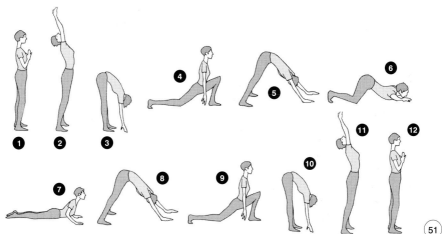

EXERCISE FOR ENERGY

ALEXANDER TECHNIQUE

The Alexander Technique (developed by Frederick Matthias Alexander in the early 1900s) focuses on creating ease of movement and improving posture. It concentrates on the relationship of the head, neck and back to help integrate and co-ordinate movements, and re-educate the body to natural posture and movement. It aims to bring the whole person back into balance, allowing the body to lengthen, energy to flow and breathing to be more efficient.

Standing tall to release tension
- Stand away from your desk, standing tall and imagine several balloons above your head, gently lengthening your spine up towards the ceiling
- Allow your feet to be firmly on the ground, hip-width apart, with your weight evenly balanced on both feet
- Gently release your knees, keeping them soft, and release any tension in your thighs
- Widen your shoulders and let your arms hang comfortably by your side
- Be aware of your head, neck and back gently supporting your body
- Keep looking straight ahead so that your chin does not tuck down
- Keep breathing at your natural rate
- Think of your pelvis in a neutral position, keeping your tailbone lengthening down
- Imagine drawing your navel back to your spine as you feel the lower abdominal muscles

EXERCISE FOR ENERGY

ALEXANDER TECHNIQUE

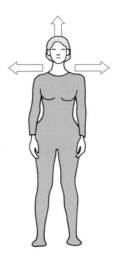

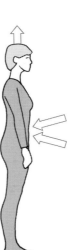

ALEXANDER TECHNIQUE

EXERCISE: ROLL DOWN AGAINST A WALL

This is a brilliant exercise to improve flexibility and strength in the spine. It releases tension in the back and aids relaxation.

It can be done against a wall or free-standing.
- Stand with your feet, foot-distance away from a wall, hip-width apart and in parallel
- Breathe in to prepare for movement and lengthen up through your spine
- As you start to breathe out, gently draw your tummy muscle in, bringing your lower abdomen towards the spine
- Allow your chin to drop forward onto your chest as you slowly roll forward, peeling the spine off the wall. Think of the spine as a wheel as you slowly peel your spine off the wall, bone by bone
- Only go as far as is comfortable, aiming eventually to reach the floor
- Breathe in as your hands reach towards the floor, allowing your arms and hands to relax down and keeping your knees soft
- Breathe out as you drop the tailbone down and rotate the pelvis slightly. Slowly, bone by bone, curl your spine back onto the wall as you come up, placing each vertebrae on the wall one by one, returning to a standing position, head last

ALEXANDER TECHNIQUE

EXERCISE: ROLL DOWN AGAINST A WALL

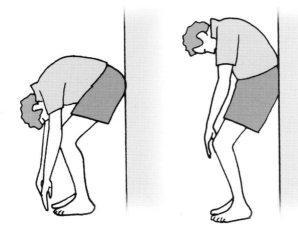

BREATHING TECHNIQUES

Remembering to breathe is, thankfully, something we do not have to do. However, **how** we breathe is important.

By breathing more efficiently we experience the following benefits:

- Improved nourishment to nerves, glands and organs
- Increased oxygen supply improves bones, teeth and hair
- The gentle expansion of the rib cage exercises the muscles between the ribs, which in turn encourages greater flexibility of the upper body
- Slow, deep breathing helps to reduce stress by reversing the stress response and calming the nerves
- Breathing deeply during exercise enhances relaxation and encourages greater ease of movement

Some breathing exercises may make you feel slightly light-headed owing to the increase in oxygen.

EXERCISE FOR ENERGY

BREATHING TECHNIQUES
RELAXED DEEP BREATHING EXERCISE

- In a standing or sitting position, gently place your hands on your lower ribs with the middle fingers just touching

- Take a deep breath, in through your nose, into the lower ribcage so you feel your fingers move slightly apart

- Breathe out through your mouth as your ribs slowly drop back down and your fingers come closer together again

- Repeat this for several breaths, breathing in through your nose and out through your mouth. You may also choose to count as you breathe, breathing in for a count of three and out for a count of three. You may find in time that you can breathe for longer, as your lungs become more familiar with relaxed, deep breathing. Breathing in for a count of 3 and out for a count of 5 will also help you relax your breathing further

EXERCISE FOR ENERGY

PERSONAL FITNESS PROGRAMME

Create your own personal fitness programme from the
following suggestions:

- Walk somewhere every day
- Choose exercise you enjoy. Exercise with friends and
  vary your activities
- Remember to gently stretch your body after activity
- Alternate strength and flexibility exercises, perhaps on
  different days of the week
- Remember that rest and recovery are vitally important
- Steadily increase duration and pace of walks
- Increase resistance of strength training
- Maintain water and food (fuel) intake
  (eg energy bars)

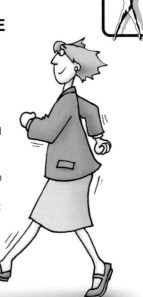

PERSONAL FITNESS PROGRAMME

Now consider the following three questions:

1. What is your **fitness** goal?
   Eg I will take the stairs every day
   instead of the lift

2. How will you start? What are the
   first steps to action?
   Eg The next time I get to the lift, I
   will carry on going and walk up the stairs

3. How will you know you have
   achieved it?
   Eg After a few days, I will start
   to feel fitter and be less out of breath
   when I reach the top of the stairs

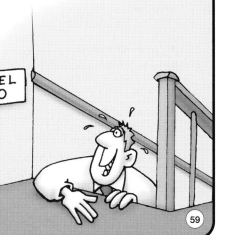

EXERCISE FOR ENERGY

ACTION PLAN

Use this space to list the personal actions you will take to make you feel fitter and more energetic.

_____   _____

_____   _____

_____   _____

_____   _____

_____   _____

_____   _____

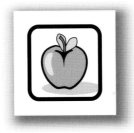

ENERGY FUEL (NUTRITION)

ENERGY FUEL (NUTRITION)

WE ARE WHAT WE EAT

What we eat has a huge impact on how we feel each day and how much energy we may have. How do you feel after eating a big meal: tired, bloated, lazy, or charged with energy, raring to go?

This section will highlight key messages about energy foods to make a difference to your health and well-being.
'We are what we eat.'

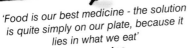

'Food is our best medicine - the solution is quite simply on our plate, because it lies in what we eat'
Hippocrates

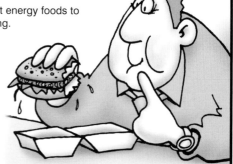

ENERGY FUEL (NUTRITION)

THE IMPORTANCE OF WATER

We need to drink sufficient water each day to maintain the energy levels in both body and brain.

The body loses some two-and-a-half litres of fluid in normal body functions daily. This needs replacing.

The thirst centre in the brain (hypothalamus) regulates both the sensation of hunger and thirst. The two are controlled separately but often your body mistakes the feeling of thirst for hunger instead. When you feel hungry, having a glass of water first can often disperse the so-called 'hunger' pangs. Water gives the body natural energy!

A note for anyone with elderly parents - The sensation of thirst in people over 70 years is very much diminished and older people often neglect to drink sufficient water, affecting the body temperature regulation.

ENERGY FUEL (NUTRITION)

THE IMPORTANCE OF WATER

Water can be absorbed immediately, helping to *kick-start* the body into action.

- Aim to drink at least two to three litres a day (eight to ten standard glasses), sipping throughout the day

- Follow the 30 minute rule and avoid drinking at meal times; it dilutes the digestive juices, delaying digestion and the absorption of nutrients

- Water at room temperature is best, but hot or cold water is fine

- Try adding a slice of lemon or fresh ginger and half a teaspoon of honey, which helps to cleanse the body of harmful toxins and stimulates the liver and kidneys as well

- If you have a headache or feel low in energy, have a glass of water first and notice the difference in how you feel

When considering other drinks, avoid caffeine in tea or coffee by trying herb tea (or Chinese green tea) in preference. They are high in vitamins and minerals, protecting the heart and lowering the blood pressure, and help to stimulate the mind and body.

ENERGY FUEL (NUTRITION)

HEALTHY SNACKS

The role of snack food is to replace and restore energy for the body to enhance learning and mental efficiency. It is important to maintain the blood sugar (glucose) level to maintain peak performance.

Some snacks (biscuits, chocolates, sweet pastries) are laden with preservatives, sugar and hidden fat, so beware!

ENERGY FUEL (NUTRITION)

HEALTHY SNACKS

Healthy snack options to consider:

- **Fruit** - only takes 20 minutes to digest, providing a quick energy source, eg apples, bananas, apricots, pears and grapes
- Try unsulphured dried fruit, eg apricots, raisins, dates, tropical fruit mixtures
- **Nuts and seeds**: almonds, brazils, cashews, hazelnuts, pumpkin seeds, sunflower seeds are high in vitamins and minerals, and contain essential fatty acids and protein
    - pumpkin seeds act as a male sexual tonic and are good for the prostate gland
    - sunflower seeds are a good energy tonic
- Try a **currant bun** or **tea cake** (150 calories) instead of a jam doughnut (250 calories)
- **Oat-based energy bars** such as flapjacks are a healthier alternative. Choose the low sugar varieties. Oats are particularly good as they contain phosphorus, which is required for brain and nerve function

The digestion of fruit is enhanced if you eat it without other food types, perhaps as a mid-morning or mid-afternoon snack. Fruit is a rich source of vitamins and minerals, and an excellent source of dietary fibre.

ENERGY FUEL (NUTRITION)

FOOD TO STIMULATE THE BRAIN

If you want to maintain peak performance and enhance learning, memory skills and brain function, consider the following tips:

- The brain is made up of 85% water, so drinking at least two litres of water a day is essential for healthy functioning of your brain cells
- Breaking-the-fast at breakfast is important for maintaining energy levels to stimulate brain function
- Processed food and foods high in fat, sugar and salt are not beneficial for brain cells, so are best avoided
- Regular meals help maintain sufficient glucose stores and iron levels for increased energy
- Remember the valuable Omega-3 fatty oils found in fish (sardines, herrings, pilchards, salmon), pumpkin seeds and nuts (walnuts, brazils, almonds, cashews)
- High energy food for the brain includes oats and brown rice. These help in the production of serotonin, an important neuro-transmitter enhancing mental and thinking skills

ENERGY FUEL (NUTRITION)

STRESS-RELIEVING FOODS

Digesting certain foods can have a stress effect on the body, which is exacerbated by the fast pace of modern life. This can increase acid production leading to heartburn, tiredness and stomach pain. The acid production is also worsened by alcohol, coffee, carbonated drinks, cheese, tobacco and sweet food (cakes, biscuits).

To create a healthier balance in the body, aim for more alkaline-based foods, eat regularly, never skipping meals, and maintain a high intake of water.

- Broccoli and green leafy vegetables - high in magnesium which soothes the nervous system. Try soya beans and bananas also
- Potassium helps conduct nerve impulses and keeps the brain's neurotransmitters working well. Try bananas, spinach, parsley and oranges
- Fruits - apples, apricots, blackcurrants
- Potatoes - soothing for the nervous system and help to neutralise body acids
- Carrots - high in zinc to boost the immune system and a powerful antioxidant
- Nuts and seeds - high in vitamins and minerals
- Almonds - alkalise the blood, help the lungs and intestines and contain essential fats
- Celery - calms the nerves
- Herbal teas - rich in vitamins and minerals

ENERGY FUEL (NUTRITION)

POWER LUNCHES

Power lunches focus on eating mainly protein food, for cellular and muscular growth.

Protein is digested slowly over a longer period of time and does not put instant demands on the digestive system, the way that a carbohydrate meal can.

It is easier for the body to digest protein alone (when combined with carbohydrate it puts unnecessary demands on the digestion and may cause the after lunch sluggish feeling!).

At lunchtime, aim to eat protein and salad, or protein and vegetables to stimulate clear thinking for the afternoon.

Aim for 1gm protein per kg body weight per day. (Beware of high protein diets as they can cause stress on the kidneys and increase the risk of osteoporosis in women, by reducing the body's ability to retain calcium.)

Protein ideas:
- Fish - helps to improve blood flow and reduce cholesterol - try sardines, mackerel, salmon, herring, tuna, trout
- Eggs
- Lean meat
- Dried and sprouted beans and pulses
- Nuts - almonds, brazils, cashews
- Soya protein and tofu

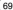

FRUIT AND VEGETABLES

Vegetables are rich in nutrients, vitamins and minerals, and easy for the body to digest. They are a good source of dietary fibre, which cleanses the digestive system.

- Dark green vegetables, eg broccoli (buy an extra bunch each week) - good for the heart, high in flavonoids
- Red peppers - high in vitamin C and carotenoids for healthy lungs and immune system
- Tomatoes - contain the pigment lycopene to help reduce the risk of cancer
- Onions - purify the blood, improve the immune system, lower blood pressure and cholesterol
- Carrots - rich in beta-carotene, good for respiratory infections, skin, eyes, blood cells
- Peas - good for digestion, high in fibre and good for the lungs

ENERGY FUEL (NUTRITION)

ENERGY FOOD

GLYCAEMIC INDEX

Food provides the energy and fuel we need for our daily activities, and provides the nutrients and minerals required to maintain the healthy functioning of our bodies.

Importance of the Glycaemic Index

The Glycaemic Index is an indicator used in carbohydrate food. It shows how quickly carbohydrate is converted into blood glucose to provide energy for the body.

If the level of carbohydrate in the food is too high, the blood sugar level can soar. This causes excess insulin to be released into fatty tissue, with the energy expenditure stored as fat in the body, thus affecting our weight.

There are two levels of Glycaemic Index foods: low and high.

ENERGY FUEL (NUTRITION)

ENERGY FOOD

GLYCAEMIC INDEX (Cont'd)

Low Glycaemic Index foods:
- Are absorbed slowly and convert glucose more steadily
- Often contain fewer calories
- Provide increased energy stores
- Make you feel full for longer, preventing snacking
- Help maintain ideal weight

Examples (aim to eat **more** of these):
Wholegrain bread, wholegrain pasta, brown rice, sweet potatoes, beans, lentils, dried fruit, most fruit and vegetables, unrefined cereals (oats)

High Glycaemic Index foods:
- Require more insulin and convert glucose quickly
- Cause a rapid surge in blood sugar levels, followed by a rapid drop
- Are often stored as fat

Examples (aim to eat **less** of these)
White bread, white pasta, pizza, white rice, sweet biscuits, cakes, processed breakfast cereals, sweetcorn, tropical fruits (bananas)

ENERGY FUEL (NUTRITION)

HOW WE EAT

Take time to eat:
- Digestion starts as soon as food enters the mouth
- Take time to chew food to allow the saliva to start breaking down the food
- Place your knife and fork down in-between mouthfuls and take time to talk, to slow down eating

Watch your position:
- To digest food the stomach and intestine need space
- Sit comfortably with your back upright (not slumped on the sofa)

Portion size:
- Beware of the man-sized meal trap!
- Women do not need to pile as much on their plates as men

When eating out:
- Try two starters or soup and a starter for a business lunch, instead of trying to eat all three courses and feeling too full afterwards

ENERGY FUEL (NUTRITION)

GOOD PRACTICE

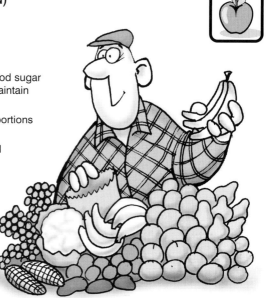

- Eat regularly; keeping your blood sugar levels constant will help you maintain your energy levels

- Remember to eat at least five portions of fruit/vegetables a day

- Aim to eat a variety of seasonal and colourful foods every day

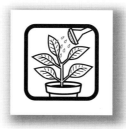

CREATING AN
ENERGETIC ENVIRONMENT

CREATING AN ENERGETIC ENVIRONMENT

VISUAL INFLUENCE

The environment around you can have a profound effect on how you feel and function and whether you feel creative, focused and relaxed. As individuals we can take on the energy of the space around us, whether at work, in our homes or gardens. If the environment around you is untidy, dirty, cluttered, etc, the sense will be reflected into your mind through your peripheral vision. You may find it harder to focus effectively on key tasks due to the many visual distractions filling the space around you.

The physical space you are in when you have creative thoughts and ideas is not necessarily at your desk. Most creative thoughts occur when you are relaxed and away from your usual work situation, eg in the shower, in the bath, taking a walk in the country.

Creating an energetic environment around you can have positive effects on your health, efficiency, enjoyment and speed of completing certain tasks.

CREATING AN ENERGETIC ENVIRONMENT

YOUR SURROUNDINGS

Think of your space around you now:

- Does it make you feel good?
- Do you have a clear desk surface in front of you? Are you hiding under a mound of papers?
- What is the view from your desk?
- What is hiding under your desk?
- How organised is your office space, filing system, storage area?
- Can you easily access information you use regularly?
- Could other people find things for you, if required?
- Would you be happy to show someone else where you work?
- Is the light directed over your work area or do you have glare from poorly positioned lights?
- If there is a lot of paper on your desk, ask yourself, *'How long have some of these pieces of paper been on my desk?'* Is it time to recycle them, file them or throw them away?
- Is it peaceful and quiet or is there lots of background noise?

CREATING YOUR IDEAL WORKSPACE

Creating your ideal workspace will depend on the space you have available, whether it is in your home, a busy open-plan work environment or private office.

Consider the following ten priorities:

1. Desk position and shape - a curved desk area is often preferred to hard, sharp lines and corners.
2. Surface of desk area - ensure your desk area allows sufficient space for your computer equipment, phone, and papers or documents you are working on.
3. Space under your desk - ensure the space under your desk is as clear as possible and not cluttered with unwanted boxes.
4. Lighting - ensure you have direct lighting on the desk area, but not providing a distracting glare onto the computer screen.

CREATING YOUR IDEAL WORKSPACE

5. Chair - adjust your chair for comfort to ensure your feet are firmly on the floor. Your low back should be supported to maintain the natural curve of the spine. If your chair doesn't have a lumbar support, you can try placing a rolled-up small towel to support your back. Adjust the height of the seat and seat angle if possible, so your hips are slightly higher than your knees. You may also wish to try a kneeling stool from a specialist back shop.

6. If you are using a computer keyboard, you should be able to rest your fingertips lightly on the keyboard with your elbows at approximately right angles (90 degrees) to the surface of the desk, with your upper arms relaxed at the side of your body. Your wrists should be straight and your forearms parallel to the desktop. (Take care not to wedge your telephone between your shoulder and your ear!)

7. Height of computer screen - adjust this to ensure your head is upright and not pushed forward or back to see the screen. The use of a document stand may also be beneficial.

8. View - be aware of the view from your desk! Can you rest your eyes by looking out of a window to focus on the distance or across to plants in the office area?

CREATING YOUR IDEAL WORKSPACE

9. Sound - if you have an office area at home or can use personal audio equipment while working, consider listening to background music to enhance creativity. Certain music has been found to be particularly effective to enhance creativity, and stimulate learning and memory. Baroque music is the same tempo as the alpha waves that the brain produces when it is in its ideal state for learning and relaxed attentiveness. Listening to certain music can encourage the brain to emit brain waves of a similar frequency, thus improving learning and concentration, eg Bach, Beethoven, Handel, Mozart (sometimes referred to as the *Mozart Effect*).

10. Consider fresh flowers and plants - these have an uplifting effect on the environment around you. They also help to remove the harmful effects on the body from computer equipment which can make people feel lethargic and tired. The harmful ions, as they are called, are found around most computers and electrical equipment, photocopiers, phones, etc. Plants help to combat the negative effects.

CREATING AN ENERGETIC ENVIRONMENT

JOURNEY TO WORK
YOUR TRAVELLING SPACE

Be aware of your journey to work:

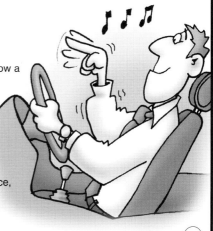

- How relaxed are you when travelling?
- Could you vary your route occasionally to allow a change of perspective?
- What would make your travelling more enjoyable and relaxing?
- What music or radio channel would help create a more relaxing or recharging environment for you?

If you travel by car, also be aware of your car space, the contents of the boot and car compartments. Again, ensure that the space works for you and is kept as tidy and organised as possible.

RECHARGING AND RELAXING SPACE AT HOME AND WORK

Creating a relaxing space in your home is also very important to help you unwind and recharge personal batteries after a busy day. You may have a favourite chair, an area you really like to sit or relax in, or an area you can escape to, to be away from busy family life.

Consider the effect of lighting, candles, music, style and positioning of chairs, pictures and artwork, etc, to help create the atmosphere that is ideal for you.

This is particularly important if you have a study or work area at home. Try to separate the home and work areas if possible, even if you just position a plant or screen to allow separation from a relaxing home area to an effective, efficient workspace.

Make your space work for you.

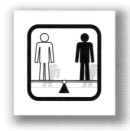

TIME FOR YOURSELF

MANAGING YOUR WORK/LIFE BALANCE

We all lead such busy lives, as we try to juggle the increasing demands of the 24 hour/7-day-a week culture of the 21st century, eg mobile phones, emails, deadlines, traffic jams, technology advances and the global economy. We are often trying to balance many tasks every day, involving work, partner, children, caring for older people, looking after pets or travelling, etc. We sometimes feel the endless jobs just never get done and that the in-tray is forever full. Maintaining a work/life balance with time for yourself is of increasing importance.

This section is about regaining the balance in your life, doing something you enjoy every day and acknowledging all the tasks that you complete. It is about finding some 'me time', time for yourself to relax and recharge your batteries. It may only be for a few moments, but it is important to grab those occasional seconds to create the energy reserves and resources you need.

HOW IS YOUR WORK/LIFE BALANCE?

Does the feeling sound familiar?

Too much to do......   Too many meetings.....   Too many jobs......
Too little time.....   Too few competent people around .....   Too........

Are you always hurrying around?

The Hurry Pattern

The hurry pattern may occur as your stress levels rise and your tolerance for waiting reduces. The following situations may be familiar to you or your colleagues!

- Restaurants where the service seems unbearably slow
- Hanging up the telephone if you are 'on hold' for more than a few seconds
- Interrupting an older relative who is speaking slowly
- The red lights which seem impossibly long
- Racing to be the first in the queue

The skill is knowing when and how to slow down!

TIME FOR YOURSELF

MONITORING YOUR PRESSURE VALVES

Understanding how you react to pressure is a key starting point in regaining time for yourself.

The Pressure Performance Stages

Consider where you are on the following table. Are you steadily reaching the crest of the wave, or travelling down the other side?

For some people the curve may be gently sloping; for others it will be a sharp peak. Know the shape of your team's curve as well as your own.

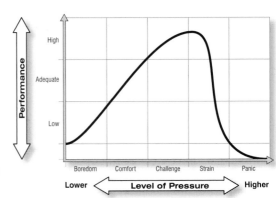

RECOGNISING SYMPTOMS OF PRESSURE

SELF

It is important to recognise the warning signs of pressure so you know when you really need to recharge the batteries.

Some pressure signs:

- Constantly tired, irritable, low energy
- Anxious, demoralised, unable to cope, depressed
- Argumentative
- Missing deadlines, making mistakes, poor concentration
- Less sociable, loss of humour
- Loss of confidence, low self-esteem
- Sleeping badly - you wake early, but find it hard to get out of bed

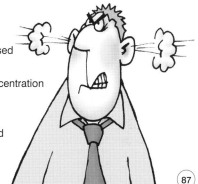

RECOGNISING SYMPTOMS OF PRESSURE

SELF AND COLLEAGUES

You may observe the following clues in colleagues, hear certain sounds or personally experience some of the feelings which can be linked to increased pressure:

SEE	Nail biting, twitching, biting of lips, excessive blinking, change in eating or drinking patterns, signs of tiredness, crying
HEAR	Slamming of doors, phones, papers or fists on desks, unusually rapid speech, drumming of fingers, emotional outbursts, swearing, uncoordinated speech, jingling of coins or keys, pen-top flicking, sighing
FEEL	Sweaty, clammy, flushed, tense, frustrated, angry, isolated, hopeless, impatient, irritable, depressed, anxious, stretched, challenged

THINKING SKILLS TO REGAIN TIME

HOW TO EXCHANGE YOUR THINKING

Pressure in our lives is often caused by how we **view** a situation, rather than the situation itself. We have a choice how we respond to difficult, challenging or stressful situations.

How you think about a situation results in certain emotions, which can cause different behaviour patterns. If you are feeling annoyed you can pass that feeling onto other people you meet. Alternatively, you may feel very positive about a situation, so you smile and look happy. This makes others working with you feel good. Remind yourself how you feel if you have an unhappy person around you.

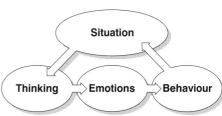

Ask yourself:

- What am I thinking?
- Is my thinking helpful and rational?
- What is a more helpful thought?

Take control of your thinking to change your emotional response and behaviour.

CREATING A SENSE OF CONTROL

Use the **3 A's model** to help control your feelings to regain a positive state.

Decide if you can   **A - A**lter
                         A - Avoid
                         A - Accept the situation that causes stress

(Source: ref Professor Stephen Palmer, Centre for Stress Management)

Or consider the **STOP strategy** to take control of your thinking.

The STOP tool   **S -** Step back
                    T - Think
                    O - Organise your thoughts
                    P - Proceed

(Source: ref W. Timothy Gallwey)

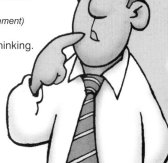

TIME FOR YOURSELF

WAYS TO RELAX

RECHARGE AND RELAX

The following pages describe simple exercises you can use to help you relax.

- Eye relaxation - around a clock face!
- Take mini breaks - 'walkabout', cross crawl exercise, figure of eight hand exercise!
- Breathing - five deep breaths (see Exercise for Energy section)

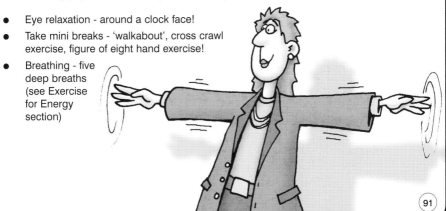

 91

WAYS TO RELAX

EYE RELAXATION

- Sit with your head squarely on your shoulders and open your eyes wide
- Keep your head still and raise your eyes to look towards the ceiling; hold this position for a slow count of five
- Roll your eyes slowly round to your right, focus on something and hold it for a slow count of five
- Keeping your head still, roll your eyes down, focus and hold for a slow count of five
- Roll your eyes to the left, focus and hold for a slow count of five
- Roll your eyes upwards again and repeat in the other direction
- Finally, close your eyes, let your head and shoulders relax and rest for a few moments

TIME FOR YOURSELF

WAYS TO RELAX

EYE RELAXATION (Cont'd)

If you are in an area where it is possible to close your eyes for the whole exercise, you may want to vary this eye relaxation. Keeping your eyes closed and head still, imagine a clock face in front of you. Move your eyes slowly to the positions of 3pm, 6pm, 9pm and 12pm. At each position take a deep breath in and out and think of the experiences listed below. Repeat the exercise moving your eyes anticlockwise.

- 3pm - take your imagination to your favourite holiday destination and imagine you are actually there
- 6pm - think of a water scene, eg a beautiful river, waterfall, seaside or fountain and swim in the water
- 9pm - think of your favourite animal or pet and imagine stroking or cuddling the animal, eg feel the soft fur of a puppy
- 12pm - think of a beautiful woodland area and take yourself high amongst the top of the trees, seeing the view all around you; or imagine you are in a beautiful garden and breathe in the scent of all the flowers

TIME FOR YOURSELF

WAYS TO RELAX

TAKE MINI BREAKS

Try getting up, moving around, going 'walkabout' for a few minutes, to refresh your mind and move your body.

You may also want to try the following two simple exercises designed by the Brain Gym, to increase your brain power by working on the left and right sides of the brain!

1.   Cross crawl exercise - similar to the front crawl in swimming!

Start by standing up and then reach forward, taking your right hand across to your left knee. Return to standing and then take your left hand towards your right knee. Continue making the movement using alternate hands at least five times to stimulate blood and oxygen flow around your body. You will be standing throughout the exercise, but leaning forwards to touch your knees.

TIME FOR YOURSELF

WAYS TO RELAX

TAKE MINI BREAKS (Cont'd)

2. Figure of eight exercise

Stretch your hands out in front of you and cross over your hands, clasping your palms gently. Bring your crossed palms towards your chest. If you have a friend nearby, ask them to point to your fingers in turn, to get you to move your fingers. This is a fun challenge as the mind tries to unravel which finger has been pointed to, which is difficult to see with fingers and hands crossed.

To encourage your mind to be more flexible and change some deep habits, try crossing your arms the unfamiliar way, brushing your teeth with the other hand or writing your name with your non-dominant hand!

Sometimes it is good to stretch your mind to do something a different way. Opening up your mind to new ideas and thoughts can result in more flexible behaviour, which allows you to take time for yourself.

TAKING ACTION

Think positively - find a more positive thought.
Take personal action - what can you yourself do to improve
the situation?

Think of a situation or task which has been challenging for
you and that you would like to change in some way.
Think of a more positive thought or action to improve
the situation and how you feel.

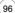

CREATING SPARE RESERVES

Do something to make a difference - what can you do personally to make more time for yourself?

- Think a positive thought as you wake up
- Choose a time each day to do the eye relaxation exercise
- Aim to move from your computer at least every 45 minutes
- Decide what would help to make your travelling more relaxed
- Identify friends you would prefer to spend time with
- Consider relaxing activities that you can do with your friends, partner, children
- Think of how you could finish work on time at least two days a week, to see the children, walk the dog, go for a swim
- Allow yourself an occasional treat, eg beauty treatment, massage, special glass of wine, Sunday afternoon siesta, visiting your favourite sports event, etc

WHAT MAKES A DIFFERENCE FOR YOU?

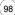

Decide what will personally make a difference for you and commit to achieving one of your key goals by a certain time. Use the **SMART** goal setting process:

S - specific and positive
M - measurable and meaningful
A - achievable
R - realistic
T - timed and targeted

Example: To introduce walking into your lifestyle, try the following SMART goal:

S - Next Saturday afternoon I will go for a walk which is beneficial for my health
M - I will monitor how far I walk in a 15 minute time period
A - I will increase the distance I walk every Saturday while keeping within my 15 minute time period
R - The maximum time I need to find is 15 minutes each Saturday
T - My target is 15 minutes each Saturday and every week I will increase the distance covered by increasing the walking pace.

Cherish the moments to relax. What would help you relax now? What simple changes can you make each day to allow a few more relaxing moments?

TIME FOR YOURSELF

CONTINGENCY AND SURVIVAL TIPS

It is useful to have some contingency plans for when the best made plans just don't quite work out.

Consider the following survival tips to provide a quick burst of energy or brief moment to recharge.

1. Drink a glass of water to provide instant energy, or eat a piece of fruit
2. Take a brief walk outside, as a fresh air break, instead of a cigarette break!
3. Breathe deeply for three long breaths in and out
4. Think of your happy memory bank and trigger those happy thoughts in your mind, to allow endorphins and happy hormones to flow in your body
5. Think of your favourite piece of music or better still, listen to it
6. Focus your eyes away from the computer screen and into the distance
7. Do some desk exercises, eg shoulder shrug, T junction, executive stretch
8. Allow yourself a lunch break or even a tea/coffee break
9. Buy a favourite magazine and read it

TIME FOR YOURSELF

RELAX

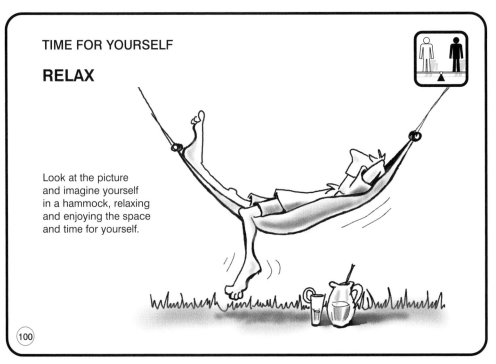

Look at the picture
and imagine yourself
in a hammock, relaxing
and enjoying the space
and time for yourself.

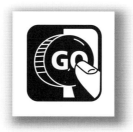

YOUR ENERGY ACTION PLAN

YOUR ENERGY ACTION PLAN

NEXT STEPS

Throughout this book we have considered ideas and techniques to improve your energy and well-being.

This last section helps you design your own energy action plan to provide the next steps on your journey to increasing energy and well-being.

For each of the sections in the book consider what would enhance your personal energy:

The Energy Factor
What is your well-being goal?
What are your energy times of the day? Are you an owl or a lark?
What are your triggers to creating endorphins and positive thoughts each day?
Have you established a bedtime sleeping routine?

Exercise for Energy
Which desk exercises will you do?
What new exercise will you try?
When can you incorporate regular energy breaks?

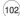

YOUR ENERGY ACTION PLAN

NEXT STEPS

Energy Fuel (Nutrition)
Which new foods are you going to try?
How will you make your snacks healthy?
Water - how much have you drunk today?
Which extra fruit and vegetables will you include each day?

Creating an Energetic Environment
How can you change your work area to be more effective for you?
What will you do to create a relaxing space at home?
What changes will you make to the space around you?

Time for Yourself
What are you going to change to allow yourself time to relax and recharge your batteries?
How are you monitoring your pressure valves?
Which contingency and survival tips are you going to try?

YOUR ENERGY ACTION PLAN

PERSONAL ENERGY ACTION MAP

Write your key ideas on the
following health map.
Or create your own unique
picture of your energy
and well-being goals.

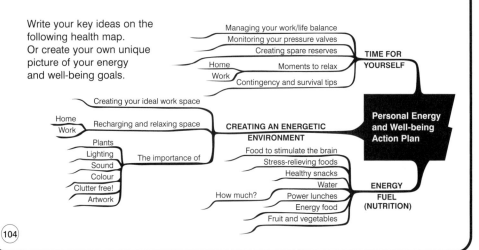

Managing your work/life balance
Monitoring your pressure valves
Creating spare reserves
Home — Moments to relax
Work — Contingency and survival tips

TIME FOR YOURSELF

Creating your ideal work space
Home
Work — Recharging and relaxing space

CREATING AN ENERGETIC ENVIRONMENT

Plants
Lighting
Sound — The importance of
Colour
Clutter free!
Artwork

Food to stimulate the brain
Stress-relieving foods
Healthy snacks
Water
How much? — Power lunches
Energy food
Fruit and vegetables

ENERGY FUEL (NUTRITION)

Personal Energy and Well-being Action Plan

PERSONAL ENERGY ACTION MAP

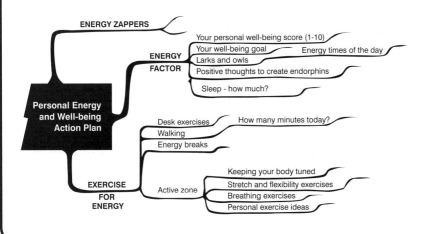

ENERGY ZAPPERS

ENERGY FACTOR
- Your personal well-being score (1-10)
- Your well-being goal — Energy times of the day
- Larks and owls
- Positive thoughts to create endorphins
- Sleep - how much?

Personal Energy and Well-being Action Plan

- Desk exercises — How many minutes today?
- Walking
- Energy breaks

EXERCISE FOR ENERGY
- Active zone
  - Keeping your body tuned
  - Stretch and flexibility exercises
  - Breathing exercises
  - Personal exercise ideas

MY PERSONAL ENERGY ENHANCERS TO CREATING POSITIVE ENERGY

Consider now what you need to do or change in your life to help enhance your energy each day. You may consider exercise tips, nutrition ideas, the space around you, time for yourself, etc.

- Can you involve friends, family or work colleagues?
- When will you start?
- Is there anything else you need to help you?

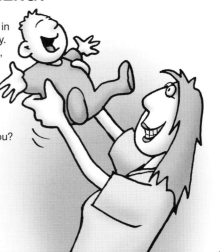

VISUALISING THE NEW ENERGETIC YOU

The visualisation technique is very useful to help bring your energy goals into action. It is powerful to use all the senses in visualising your goal. It helps to bring your goal 'alive' so you can imagine yourself actually achieving your desired goal.

- What will it look like? *The visual representation of your goal*
- What will you hear or what will people be saying? *The sounds or positive comments people may make*
- What will you feel? *The feelings and sensations you may experience*
- What will it taste like? *Even consider the tastes, smells or aromas you may experience*

The trick is to make it as colourful and realistic as possible with all the appropriate thoughts and feelings going through your body as if you are really enjoying your energy goal **now**.

FURTHER READING

Brain Gym, Exercises for Business   Dennison, Dennison and Teplitz
Published by Edu-Kinesthetics, California
ISBN 0942143035

The Mozart Effect   Don Campbell
Published by Hodder and Stoughton, London
ISBN 0340824379

Body Control the Pilates Way   Lynne Robinson and Gordon Thomas
Published by Pan Books
ISBN 0330369458

About the Author

Gillian Burn, MSc in Exercise and Health

Gillian is Director of Health Circles Ltd, providing training and consultancy services focusing on improving health and quality of life for individuals and companies nationwide. Her background is in the health field, spanning over 25 years and covering nursing, midwifery and health visiting. Gillian is a master practitioner in Neuro-Linguistic Programming (NLP) and Time Line Therapy® which she uses in workshops with companies and coaching for individuals. Her workshops focus on training people to use their minds and bodies to increase energy and performance. This includes nutrition and exercise advice, understanding the mind and body connection, creating balance in our lives, and techniques to increase creativity and effectiveness.

She is a licensed instructor with Tony Buzan for training in Mind Mapping® techniques and has trained in speed reading and memory techniques, and also runs training courses in these areas. In addition, Gillian is a trainer in Body Control Pilates Exercise. Gillian aims to practise what she preaches! She rows on the River Thames and enjoys swimming, walking, yoga and pilates.

Contact

Gillian can be contacted at: +44 (0) 1628 666 069 and via www.healthcircles.co.uk

THE MANAGEMENT POCKETBOOK SERIES

Pocketbooks

360 Degree Feedback
Appraisals
Assertiveness
Balance Sheet
Business Planning
Business Writing
Call Centre Customer Care
Career Transition
Coaching
Communicator's
Competencies
Controlling Absenteeism
Creative Manager's
C.R.M.
Cross-cultural Business
Cultural Gaffes
Customer Service
Decision-making
Developing People
Discipline
Diversity
E-commerce
Emotional Intelligence
Employment Law
Empowerment

Energy and Well-being
Facilitator's
Flexible Workplace
Handling Complaints
Icebreakers
Impact & Presence
Improving Efficiency
Improving Profitability
Induction
Influencing
International Trade
Interviewer's
I.T. Trainer's
Key Account Manager's
Leadership
Learner's
Manager's
Managing Budgets
Managing Cashflow
Managing Change
Managing Difficult Participants
Managing Recruitment
Managing Upwards
Managing Your Appraisal
Marketing

Meetings
Mentoring
Motivation
Negotiator's
Networking
NLP
Openers & Closers
People Manager's
Performance Management
Personal Success
Positive Mental Attitude
Presentations
Problem Behaviour
Problem Solving
Project Management
Resolving Conflict
Reward
Sales Excellence
Salesperson's
Self-managed Development
Starting In Management
Strategy
Stress
Succeeding at Interviews
Talent Management

Teambuilding Activities
Teamworking
Telephone Skills
Telesales
Thinker's
Time Management
Trainer Standards
Trainer's
Training Evaluation
Training Needs Analysis
Virtual Teams
Vocal Skills

Pocketsquares

Great Training Robbery

Pocketfiles

Trainer's Blue Pocketfile of
Ready-to-use Activities

Trainer's Green Pocketfile of
Ready-to-use Activities

Trainer's Red Pocketfile of
Ready-to-use Activities

19.09.07

ORDER FORM

Your details

Name _____

Position _____

Company _____

Address _____

_____

_____

Telephone _____

Fax _____

E-mail _____

VAT No. (EC companies) _____

Your Order Ref _____

Please send me:

		No. copies
The Energy & Well-being	Pocketbook	
The _____	Pocketbook	
The _____	Pocketbook	
The _____	Pocketbook	

Order by Post

MANAGEMENT POCKETBOOKS LTD

LAUREL HOUSE, STATION APPROACH,
ALRESFORD, HAMPSHIRE SO24 9JH UK

Order by Phone, Fax or Internet
Telephone: +44 (0)1962 735573
Facsimile: +44 (0)1962 733637
E-mail: sales@pocketbook.co.uk
Web: www.pocketbook.co.uk

Customers in USA should contact:
Management Pocketbooks
2427 Bond Street, University Park, IL 60466
Telephone: 866 620 6944 Facsimile: 708 534 7803
E-mail: mp.orders@ware-pak.com
Web: www.managementpocketbooks.com

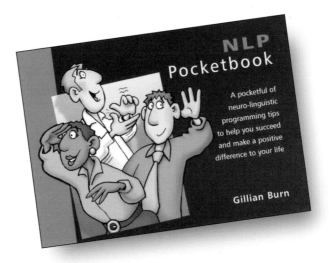

Another title by Gillian Burn in the Pocketbook Series

(see previous page for full listing)